The Support of Cedarwood Essential Oils

Benefits, Properties, Applications, Studies & Recipes

by Ann Sullivan

Published in USA by:

Ann Sullivan
217 N. Seacrest Blvd #9
Boynton Beach
FL 33425

© Copyright 2015

ISBN-13: ISBN-13: 978-1544738727
ISBN-10: ISBN-10: 1544738722

Table of Contents

Introduction

What are essential oils and how might they be used for therapeutic purposes?

Essential oils are ultra-potent oils extracted from plants and flowers that have been utilized in medicine for centuries. Presently, they are most commonly used to supplement pharmaceutical medication, but they can also be an effective alternative to pharmaceuticals in the event that there is no access to them. Before dismissing essential oils as a means to support the body's natural defenses against injury and illness, take a look at the historical evidence of the oils' medicinal competence in practice. The average age-old medical text will demonstrate that essential oils, herbs, and plenty of other natural ingredients have, for thousands of years, successfully enhanced immune function to meet and defeat any number of ailments and injuries. Though traditional medicine is considered "alternative" now, it was once the gold standard. Perhaps it still should be, as these natural age-tested remedies can fortify the body's defenses against everything from simple maladies, like headaches, cuts, and bruises to serious diseases, like cancer.

Essential oils are deemed "essential," because the oils are composed of the "essence" of the plant. The difference between essential oils and other oils – like olive oil or vegetable oil, for instance – is that essential oils have high volatility and reduced fixation, which results in faster evaporation, enabling their popular use in aromatherapy. Even at high temperatures, olive and vegetable oils do not evaporate.

Essential oils are especially necessary when it comes to a major natural or man-made disaster or potential viral outbreak. In these dire situations, people may not have quick access to their standard pharmaceutical supply; so essential oils, along with other alternative medicines, will be the go-to health aids in the case of social collapse, viral outbreak, or devastating natural disaster. When medical access is unavailable, alternatives to our modern-day standard are the only chance we have to keep pathogens at bay.

Most people do not realize that they already use essential oils every day. They are in perfumes, shampoos, soaps, and ointments; they are even used in furniture polish. Why are they found in so many aromatic products? Well, because essential oils are super concentrated aromatic liquids, so their scent is remarkably strong. Let us put this into perspective: to steam tea, use a few leaves of peppermint or juniper; to produce a single ounce of essential oil, five whole pounds of peppermint or juniper leaves are required. Some sources claim that to produce twelve pounds of essential oil would necessitate an acre of peppermint, juniper, or any other oil being produced en masse. Unlike vegetable oil, you do not often find concentrated therapeutic-grade essential oils sold in bulk; instead the oils are often sold in easily carried small, dark bottles, perfect for the GOOD bag (Get Out Of Dodge). That is exactly what this book is aiming to help people plan for – getting out of dodge with the most vital of essential oils intact, in particular a good supply of Cedarwood essential oil.

Why Cedarwood, you ask? Well, in order to get quickly up to speed on this most essential of oils, below we have provided a condensed synopsis of Cedarwood, after which we will outline in greater detail the oil's history, properties, and common therapeutic uses, so that you – the consumer – might have a better understanding of the oil's benefits and applications. We have even provided supportive remedies for pure Cedarwood, as well as blended recipes that incorporate the valuable oil. Chapter 3 will further detail past scientific research on Cedarwood essential oil.

Now, let us get down to it – **Essential Oil 101: The Basics of Cedarwood.**]

Summary: Cedarwood has been used in Tibetan, Egyptian, and Sumerian tradition and has been considered valuable for such a lengthy amount of time that it has even been documented in the Bible. Juniperus virginiana, a species of Cedarwood, is now commonly found in North America.

With the largest amount of sesquiterpenes amongst essential oils, Cedarwood stimulates cellular oxygen and circulation, which helps the body release toxins. This makes Cedarwood exceptional when it comes to supporting the body's defenses against skin and hair damage.

Description: Cedarwood oil is commonly extracted through steam distillation. The wood is most often used. The oil is clear in color, medium in consistency, and has a somewhat strong, fresh, woody scent.

Uses: Beyond those applications previously mentioned, additional uses for Cedarwood essential oil include supporting the body's defenses against arthritis, acne, cystitis, dermatitis, bronchitis, coughing, dandruff, hair loss, arteriosclerosis, tuberculosis, water retention, skin conditions, eczema, psoriasis, cellulite, urinary infections, and sleep issues. When it comes to mood and emotion, Cedarwood can help relieve fear, anxiety, nerves, or stress.

Properties: Antioxidant, antiseptic, antibacterial, anti-inflammatory, antispasmodic, antifungal, analgesic, astringent, repellant, sedative, expectorant, emmenagogue, and diuretic

Application: Use neat or undiluted. Apply topically, inhale directly, or diffuse.

Safety Precautions: Do not take internally. If pregnant, use with caution. Cedarwood is safe for children 24 months or older.

Fun facts: Cedarwood is derived from "kedron," the Arabic word for "power."

Cedarwood seems to hold spiritual power in Egyptian culture, as it was used specifically to embalm the dead. It was also spiritually powerful to the Native Americans. The Cherokee traditionally wore a small medicine bag, containing a piece of Cedarwood, around the neck to ward off evil spirits.

Chapter 1:
Benefits of Cedarwood Essential Oil

Cedarwood oil offers a number of therapeutic benefits; but you may be wondering what these benefits are. In this chapter, we'll take a closer look at the history of Cedarwood and its many uses.

Cultivation of Cedarwood

There are many species of Cedarwood, and quite a few are used in the making of essential oils. Differing species sometimes possess different qualities or properties. This book will examine those of Juniperus virginiana, as this species is used by several manufacturers of Cedarwood essential oil.

Juniperus virginiana is native to the eastern region of North America, running across southeast Canada down to the Gulf of Mexico. The juniper species is related to the Rocky Mountain Juniper and the Ashe Juniper, which are prevalent in western regions of North America.

The Juniperus virginiana is a coniferous evergreen. The tree grows slowly and sometimes amounts to nothing more than a small bush when planted in limited soil. However, in cases of favorable environmental conditions, the dense evergreen can grow from 16' – 66' tall with a narrow trunk, 12" – 39" in diameter. The tree's leaves are either sharp like needles when young (up to 3 years old) or long and scaly when mature, while the reddish bark is coarse and can be peeled off in strips. The tree produces cones which have deep bluish purple seeds like berries; these are coated in a white wax that can be scraped off. Often 1 – 3 seeds grow per cone and are pollinated after 6 months, often sprouting on separate trees than the seed cones. The pollen is shed in late winter, pollinating the seed cones. The seeds are known as juniper berries and are prominent nutrition in the diet of local birds; birds which are responsible for distributing the seeds across North America and spreading the growth of the Juniperus virginiana.

Though the Juniperus virginiana is already a sub-species, further division occurs among the subspecies, turning out two varieties of Juniperus virginiana – the virginiana variety and the silicicola variety. The virginiana variety is also known as the red cedar, or eastern juniper, and grows from the far east of Maine to the west of South

Dakota. It even grows as far south as northern Florida. The bark of this variety is reddish, the leaves are acute at the crest, and the cones are larger. The silicicola variety is also known as the red cedar or sand juniper. These grow along the coast of North Carolina into central Florida and over to southeast Texas. The bark of this variety is orange, the leaves are blunt at the crest, and the cones are smaller.

Often prevalent across pastures, prairies, limestone hills, and especially near construction sites and highways, the Juniperus virginiana is not all that friendly. In fact, it is known as an invasive species because it populates, erodes, and often damages the land upon which it has invaded. What is more, it is an old invader, one of the longest living species among the pioneers, even living as long as 850 years, and infecting nearby apple orchards with what is known as cedar-apple rust disease. The trees span widely, due to their broad branch bases, and block out the sun so that plants and grass cannot thrive. Furthermore, the species' needles increase the soil's pH levels, reducing nutrients and producing an alkaline soil which prohibits plants from absorbing the soil's limited nutrients. In essence, this species destroys grasslands, so the trees are often cut or burnt down to prevent this. However, the fact that the Juniper virginiana burns easily can be a double-edged sword, as this tends to promote rapid wildfire, particularly when droughts occur. This is why the Juniper virginiana are often deemed an invasive species, even in regions where the tree is native.

A History of Cedarwood

The ancient Egyptians and Sumerians commonly used Cedarwood that was cultivated in the western and northern mountain ranges located in the Middle East. This variety was known as the Cedar of Lebanon and the ancient forests that produced the once popular cedar are now almost completely razed. None of the Cedarwood available in modern day is derived from this species. The ancient Egyptians however, highly valued this specific Cedarwood species for its sacred applications. In fact, they used it to embalm the dead, in order to drive away insects, as the large amount of cedrol in this species induces strong anti-pesticide properties. The oil was also used by the Sumerians as a paint base.

Called "Chansha," or "redwood," by the Lakota Native Americans, the Juniperus virginiana species is incorrectly termed a "cedar," or "red cedar," names that are refuted by the American Joint Committee on Horticultural Nomenclature, being that the tree is NOT a cedar, but a juniper. The incorrect title however, has stuck and thus, Cedarwood essential oil is often extracted from this juniper tree.

The wood from this tree has long been used in the making of fence posts, as it is durable, light, and rot-resistant. The anti-pesticide qualities of its fragrance also makes it ideal in the creation of armoires, or chests for clothing, as the aroma of the wood deters moths. The

Native Americans found many uses for the juniper tree, including marking off hunting territories designated for particular tribes. This caused French traders to name the Louisiana city Baton Rouge, after the color of these markings; "Baton Rouge" in French means "red stick." The heartwood was used to create bows and up until the 1940s, pencils were also largely produced from the heartwood, though nowadays incense-cedar is primarily used for this purpose.

The wood and leaves of the Juniperus virginiana are used in the making of the Cedarwood essential oil. This essential oil is composed of a large amount of cedrol, which is toxic, thus it must not be taken internally, although the cones from the tree are sometimes utilized to flavor gin.

The oil was also used by the Native Americans and was so popular amongst the Ojibwa tribe that it ranked amongst their four sacred medicines, alongside sweet grass, white sage, and tobacco. They believed it purified the spirit and would use it in prayer and during spiritual rituals.

The Dust Bowl during the 1930s saw an increase in Juniperus virginiana cultivation, as farmers benefited from the juniper "shelterbelts" shielding the wind across the Great Plains. As the species is tolerant of rocky or otherwise tough soil, drought, cold temperatures, and other adverse conditions, they can be cultivated tightly in places where other trees cannot grow, producing a quite effective wind block. Nowadays, eastern junipers are often used as Christmas trees throughout the Ozarks and Missouri.

Cedarwood oil is often used in the present day to refresh the scent of furniture, repel insects, and to scent candles, sprays, soaps, and floor polish. The oil has also been shown to have bacterial and fungicidal properties.

Chemical Components

In order to generate the essential oil from the Juniperus virginiana, the wood must be steam distilled. This results in the oil's key chemical components, which are primarily cedrol and cedrene. The odor of the oil is due in part to these chemicals. They are also often isolated and used in combination with other chemicals to produce different fragrances in the chemical industry.

Main Properties of Cedarwood Essential Oil

Along with the properties previously mentioned in the introduction, Cedarwood oil possesses antioxidant, antiseptic, antibacterial, anti-inflammatory, antispasmodic, antifungal, analgesic, astringent, repellant, sedative, expectorant, emmenagogue, and diuretic properties. With such a versatile range, Cedarwood is well equipped to fight off any pathogen in the body.

Cedarwood, as mentioned, is composed primarily of cedrol and cedrene. These components are what instill the enormously beneficial properties within Cedarwood essential oil. We will outline these properties below.

Antioxidant

Anything high in antioxidants – whether fruit, beans, or essential oils – is a powerful advocate for the body. Antioxidants protect against free radicals and repair their damage. What are free radicals? Free radicals are destructive chemicals that invade the body, produced by substances both inside and out. Some free radicals (or oxidants) form through normal bodily reactions, like inflammation, metabolism, and aerobic respiration. Other free radicals form outside the body, but enter it due to exposure. These include harmful pollutants, toxins, smoking, drinking alcohol, X-rays, and UV rays just to name a few. Although our bodies produce their own antioxidants, these often become damaged as we grow older; thus, introducing antioxidants into our bodies allows these nutrients and enzymes to assist in chemical reactions which destroy the oxidants or free radicals. Cedarwood essential oil is a moderate antioxidant, aiming to detox the body of free radicals that lead to disease.

Antifungal

Cedarwood essential oil possesses antifungal properties which help protect against wood fungi and mildew.

Antiseptic

The antiseptic and disinfectant properties of Cedarwood essential oil can be reaped topically, applied directly to wounds, or even through burning; the smoke from the oil may help destroy airborne germs. Internal use will help keep the wounds from becoming infections, while external use will inhibit tetanus.

Antibacterial

Cedarwood's antibacterial properties make it a powerful protectant against diseases produced by bacteria, such as oral, digestive, and urinary tract bacterial infection. What is great is that, unlike some prescription drugs, Cedarwood has no ill effects on bodily health, or on the healthy natural flora that exists within the stomach and intestines.

Anti-inflammatory

External or internal inflammation can be reduced through the use of Cedarwood essential oil. For instance, if a patient has swollen fingers from arthritis, or a swollen knee from an injury, application of Cedarwood essential oil may decrease irritation or redness, while also soothing the pain that accompanies inflammation.

Antispasmodic

The antispasmodic properties of Cedarwood essential oil make it beneficial to such surgical processes as colonoscopy, gastroscopy, and intra-luminal-applied double-contrast barium enema.

Analgesic

As an analgesic, Cedarwood relieves pain, acting on the central nervous system to inhibit inflammation and relieve pain receptor sensation.

Astringent

An astringent is a chemical compound that shrinks body tissues, which means it can aid skin issues and irritations. Cedarwood essential oil benefits everything from skin to gums and muscles to intestines. As an astringent, Cedarwood is an anti-agent, combating muscle loss through its ability to strengthen.

Sedative

As a sedative, Cedarwood sedates and calms by reducing anxiety, excitement, and irritability. Though sedatives alone do not alleviate pain, they do calm the patient, making them less stressed and more compliant.

Expectorant

Throat or respiratory infections can be relieved through the use of Cedarwood essential oil. Acting as an expectorant, Cedarwood breaks up and helps destroy the phlegm and mucus buildup that accompanies sinuses or respiratory infections. Inflamed throat and lungs can also be relieved by the use of this oil.

Emmenagogue

An emmenagogue is a menstrual stimulant for those with irregular menses. Cedarwood regulates hormones, which means that this emmenagogue can also delay and/or reduce the symptoms of menopause, which include hormonal and mood imbalance.

Diuretic

If looking to lose water weight and reduce blood pressure, Cedarwood essential oil is a weight loss enhancing agent. The oil stimulates urination, promoting not only the loss of water weight, but the loss of fats, uric acid, sodium, and other body toxins.

Common Medicinal Uses

With a history of use in skincare, Cedarwood primarily promotes healthy skin; however, it has a host of other applications. Below are a few more ways in which Cedarwood essential oil can play an active role in the body's overall health.

Skin Issues

With its antibacterial and antifungal properties Cedarwood essential oil promotes healthy, glowing skin by supporting the body's natural defenses against dry or chapped skin, eczema, dermatitis, acne, and a litany of other skin issues. The oil combats bacterial growth while promoting sebum secretion balance within the body. The oil's disinfectant properties also allow for a clean healing process for any skin condition, or wound, and protects against scarring.

Hair Care

Cedarwood essential oil invokes strength, health, and shine in hair follicles, and is often used as a moisturizing hair tonic. The oil also effectively combats dandruff and hair loss, so a drop or two in your shampoo can help eliminate this issue.

Losing Weight

Those who need a boost to lose unwanted weight can use Cedarwood topically, as it has been shown to reduce water retention. This will eliminate bloating and cut out that bit of extra water weight, and also help remove toxins in the body and excess fat. The increased urinary function also reduces the chances of urinary tract infections.

Insomnia

Cedarwood essential oil can target insomnia and other sleep disorders. The calming effect of Cedarwood can help the body relax and can ease the sleepless into sleep. Those suffering from insomnia should diffuse Cedarwood essential oil in their bedroom, or place a drop or two on their linens. Adults and children alike can enjoy a faster, deeper, sounder sleep through the use of lavender oil.

Aiding Menstruation & Menopause

Women can benefit from administering Cedarwood if they commonly experience painful, or irregular periods, or unpleasant menopausal effects. Applying Cedarwood can help young women become regular, relieve painful menstrual cramps, and combat unpleasant attributes of menopause, by better maintaining hormonal balance.

Insect Repellant

You do not have to be covered in a sticky bug spray to keep the mosquitoes at bay; Cedarwood oil is a match for even the peskiest of bugs. Whether diffused in the buggy infested area, or applied topically with a few drops in a favorite skin cream, the strong insecticidal properties will stave off the bugs and will smell great doing it. It is also used to keep bugs and other pests from eating at crops.

Respiratory Issues

Respiratory issues, such as pneumonia, bronchitis, asthma, and tuberculosis can all be supported with Cedarwood essential oil. This is because Cedarwood essential oil enables more oxygen to flow into the lungs by dilating the blood vessels.

Anxiety, Stress & Depression

The scent of Cedarwood has been shown to relieve anxiety, soothe emotion, and calm nerves. The natural sedative eases anxiety, mental fatigue, nervousness, and exhaustion. If feeling stressed, combat negative emotions, or head them off through an essential oil application, whether diffused in aromatherapy practices or topically applied.

Safety Precautions & Common Applications

Safety

Some adverse effects may evolve when using pure essential oils. Some essential oils should not be used when pregnant for example. Allergic reactions may occur, especially when applied topically. Always administer an allergy test before committing fully to topical application. When used with other medications, essential oils may react negatively. If on any current prescription medications or chronic illness is present, such as high blood pressure, epilepsy, or liver disease, then researching the effects of essential oils against personal medical history will eliminate any potentially problems.

Cedarwood has not been approved by the FDA for internal consumption, so do not take orally. Use neat or diluted. You can apply topically, inhale directly, or diffuse. If pregnant, use with caution. Cedarwood is safe for children 24 months or older.

Blends

Oftentimes, essential oils are manufactured as blends of several pure oils. For instance, a Protective Oil Blend is a mix of cinnamon, clove, rosemary, and eucalyptus. This blend can be used to boost the immune system to help support the body's defenses against colds, viruses, and flus. The downside to blends is that the more oils added to the mix, the higher the probability a patient may react negatively to the blend if he/she is prone to allergies. There is also the possibility of phototoxicity when working with blends.

Regardless of these possible effects, essential oils are a viable option for supporting the body's defenses against a number of conditions. Those looking to enhance the maintenance of their own personal health, or that of their families, should become educated on the uses of essential oils, their natural remedies, and the methods of application. Only then can we begin building a kit of essential oils for survival.

Chapter 2:
Recipes for Cedarwood
Essential Oil

In this chapter, we will offer various recipes for Cedarwood essential oil, both for pure Cedarwood applications and blends. For pure supportive remedies, we have provided the appropriate application and dosage to help the body's natural function address specific ailments, from acne to water retention. When it comes to blends, herbalists and aromatherapists often combine Cedarwood essential oil with lavender, bergamot, rose, benzoin, rosemary, cypress, neroli, cinnamon, juniper, frankincense, lemon, jasmine, and lime. We will offer some fantastic supportive blending options in the second half of this chapter.

Pure Supportive Remedies

Acne

Enhance the body's natural ability to clear acne by diluting 2 drops of Cedarwood essential oil in 4-5 drops of fractionated coconut oil and applying the combo to the affected area twice daily. Suggested application is before and after showering.

Anxiety

To relieve anxiety, place 1 drop of Cedarwood essential oil into the palm and rub hands together. Place the hand over nose and mouth and inhale. Apply topically across the brow, or diffuse throughout your home, to relieve tension and stress.

Asthma

Combat asthma and open up airways; apply Cedarwood undiluted, topically by massaging over the chest during an asthma attack. Diffuse throughout the home or inhale directly to help stave off attacks.

Bladder Infection

Support the body's natural defenses against bladder infection by applying Cedarwood topically. Massage the oil undiluted, over the bladder and kidneys 3 times daily.

Calming

Calm anger, stress, or nerves by diffusing Cedarwood

essential oil throughout the home. Apply topically in a full-body massage.

Congestion

Clear congestion by applying undiluted Cedarwood topically, massaging it over the affected area and into the reflex points of the feet. Inhale the oil directly for nasal congestion.

Cough

Relieve coughing by applying undiluted Cedarwood topically, massaging it over the throat, chest, and back, as well as into the reflex points of the feet. Diffuse throughout the home to help relieve family members with respiratory issues, and help protect those who are healthy.

Dandruff

As an antifungal, Cedarwood essential oil balances the skin's pH levels and soothes dryness and irritation. Eliminate dandruff by applying directly to the scalp, or add a drop or two to your shampoo and use as normal.

Eczema

Clear up eczema by applying Cedarwood topically to the affected area. Those with sensitive skin should dilute with a carrier oil.

Grounding

To help keep grounded, place 1 drop of Cedarwood essential oil into the palm and rub hands together. Place hand over nose and mouth and inhale. Apply topically, massaging the oil into the reflex points of the feet.

Kidney Support

Support the body's natural defenses against kidney issues by applying undiluted Cedarwood essential oil topically, massaging it over the affected area, 3 times daily.

Loneliness

To help stave off loneliness, place 1 drop of Cedarwood essential oil into the palm and rub hands together. Place hand over nose and mouth and inhale. Apply topically, massaging the oil over the heart.

Moths

Keep moths at bay by applying a drop of Cedarwood essential oil to a cotton ball and setting it on a closet shelf, or into storage cartons – wherever an infestation of moths may be problematic. Apply oil every 6 months, or as needed.

Psoriasis

Cedarwood can be used to support the body's natural defenses against psoriasis. Apply Cedarwood essential oil undiluted directly to the affected area twice daily.

Skin Issues

Cedarwood can be applied to all sorts of skin conditions. Apply Cedarwood essential oil directly to the affected area, or dilute for sensitive skin. You can also add a couple of drops to bathwater, or massage into the reflex points of the feet.

Stress

Combat stress by steaming 2 drops of Cedarwood essential oil in a pan of water, remove the steaming pan from the stove, pour into a bowl, place a towel over head and inhale. Place a drop onto the shirt collar for portable stress relief, diffuse in the home, or apply topically to the chest, the top of the head, and the reflex points of the feet.

Tension

Same applications as for "stress." Simply apply undiluted Cedarwood topically, massaging it into the affected area.

Urinary Infection

Support the body's natural defenses in eliminating urinary tract infections by massaging Cedarwood into the soles of the feet, over the kidneys, urethra, and bladder. Place 3-4 drops in a sitz bath and soak in it for 10-15 minutes.

Water Retention

To reduce water retention, apply undiluted Cedarwood essential oil topically, massaging over the kidney, bladder, and into the reflex points of the feet twice daily.

Blends

Aches/Pains

Ingredients

4 drops Peppermint Essential Oil

3 drops Oregano Essential Oil

2 drops Lavender Essential Oil

2 drops Cedarwood Essential Oil

1 Tbsp. Carrier Oil

Directions

To relieve aches and pains, place all ingredients into a small bowl or container and blend thoroughly. Apply topically, massaging gently into affected area.

Comfort Massage Oil

Ingredients

2 drops Rosemary Essential Oil

2 drops Cedarwood Essential Oil

2 drops Pine Essential Oil

4 drops Helichrysum Essential Oil

4 drops German Chamomile Oil

1-ounce Jojoba Oil

Directions

For a comforting massage oil blend, combine all ingredients in a small jar or bowl, blending well. Apply topically in a full-body massage.

Fatigue Fix

Ingredients

4 drops Spruce Essential Oil

4 drops Bay Leaf Essential Oil

6 drops Cedarwood Essential Oil

2 ounces Sweet Almond Oil

Directions

To boost energy and combat fatigue, combine all ingredients in a small jar or bowl, blending well. Apply topically in a full-body massage or target fatigued areas, like the lower back and legs.

Hair & Scalp Health

Ingredients

4 drops Cedarwood Essential Oil

4 drops Lemongrass Essential Oil

4 drops Lavender Essential Oil

4 drops Peppermint Essential Oil

8 drops Rosemary Verbenone Oil

1-ounce Jojoba Oil

Directions

To support the health of hair and scalp, combine all ingredients in a small jar or bowl, blending well. Apply topically, working the formula into wet hair and scalp. Wash out with shampoo as normal.

Osteoarthritis

Ingredients

4 drops Cedarwood Essential Oil

5 drops Cypress Essential Oil

8 drops Black Pepper Essential Oil

13 drops Ginger Essential Oil

2 Tbsps. Almond Oil

Directions

To help relieve the pain and swelling caused by osteoarthritis, combine all ingredients in a small bowl, blending well. Apply topically, massaging into the affected area.

Relaxing Massage Blend

Ingredients

2 drops Roman Chamomile Essential Oil

3 drops Cedarwood Essential Oil

3 drops Anise Essential Oil

3 drops Neroli Essential Oil

4 drops Orange Essential Oil

15 ml Carrier Oil

Directions

For a relaxing massage oil blend, combine all ingredients in a small jar or bowl, blending well. Apply topically in a full-body massage.

Respiratory Stimulant

Ingredients

2 drops Eucalyptus Essential Oil

2 drops Cedarwood Essential Oil

4 drops Juniper Berry Essential Oil

4 drops Frankincense Essential Oil

1-ounce Carrier Oil

Directions

To stimulate or support the respiratory system, combine all ingredients in a small jar or bowl, blending well. Apply topically to the chest, massaging in a clockwise motion.

Sensual Massage Oil

Ingredients

2 drops Clary Sage Essential Oil

2 drops Cedarwood Essential Oil

1 drop Orange Essential Oil

20 drops Jojoba Oil

2 ounces Sunflower Oil

Directions

For a sensual massage oil blend, combine all ingredients in a small jar or bowl, blending well. Apply topically in a full-body massage.

Chapter 3:
Cedarwood Essential Oil Studies

Many studies have been done on essential oils to discover and prove their therapeutic qualities. In the case of Cedarwood studies, many of the properties attributed to the essential oil (noted in this book and elsewhere) are quite often validated through the scientific research of accredited universities and published by accredited scientific journals. In this chapter, we will discuss a small portion of these studies. It is important to note that research on essential oils is constant and evolving. Keep up with any recent research, as it may turn up even further valuable uses of these miracle oils.

Study 1 – Antibacterial Properties

In this study, available on PubMed, the antibacterial effects of Cedarwood essential oil on oral health were examined, with the following results: "To study the antibacterial activity of nine commercially available essential oils against Streptococcus mutans in vitro and to compare the antibacterial activity between each material...Cinnamon oil showed highest activity against Streptococcus mutans followed by lemongrass oil and Cedarwood oil...Cinnamon oil, lemongrass oil, Cedarwood oil, clove oil and eucalyptus oil exhibit antibacterial property against S. mutans."

Streptococcus mutans is an oral bacterium which causes cavities and tooth decay. Cedarwood was among 9 essential oils tested against this strain of bacteria and was found to be one of the most powerful in inhibiting S.mutans. This suggests that Cedarwood has potential in controlling oral infection-producing yeasts and bacteria.

Reference:
http://www.ncbi.nlm.nih.gov/pubmed/22430697]

Study 2 – Insect Repellent

In this study published by the *Journal of Parasitology Research*, the repellent effects of a Cedarwood essential oil species were examined, with the following results: "Essential oils of eight plants, selected after an ethnobotanical survey conducted in Bukusu community in Bungoma County, western Kenya (Tagetes minuta, Tithonia diversifolia, Juniperus procera, Solanecio mannii, Senna didymobotrya, Lantana camara, Securidaca longepedunculata, and Hoslundia opposita), were initially screened (at two doses) for their repellence against brown ear tick, Rhipicephalus appendiculatus...The results provide scientific rationale for traditional use of raw products of these plants in controlling livestock ticks by the Bukusu community and lay down some groundwork for exploiting partially refined products such as essential oils of these plants in protecting cattle against infestations with R. appendiculatus."

The Rhipicephalus appendiculatus, or brown ear tick, is a prominent pest native to tropical Africa. These ticks are vectors of pathogens, transmitting both animal and human diseases, such as Lyme disease, East Coast fever, Crimean-Congo hemorrhagic fever, and anaplasmosis, among many others. To top it off, when they bite, a neurotoxin is injected, resulting in tick paralysis.

Needless to say, controlling the population of R.appendiculatus is essential to protect not only cattle, but humans as well, against the possibility of spreading these diseases. Like most Cedarwood species, Juniperus procera showed repellent activity against the brown ear tick, making it potentially beneficial in the control of the tick population amongst livestock.

Reference:
http://www.ncbi.nlm.nih.gov/pubmed/24693417]

http://www.ncbi.nlm.nih.gov/pmc/articles/PMC3945150/pdf/JPR2014-434506.pdf]

Study 3 – Anti-mildew/Antifungal Properties

In this study available on PubMed, the anti-mildew and antifungal effects of Cedarwood essential oil species on wood decay were examined, with the following results: "In this study, anti-mildew and anti-wood-decay fungal activities of the leaf and fruits essential oil and its constituents from Juniperus formosana were evaluated in vitro against seven mildew fungi and four wood decay fungi, respectively."

This study aimed to assess the efficacy of Juniperus formosana, a Cedarwood oil originating from China, in preventing mildew and fungal wood decay. The study identified the main compounds responsible for anti-mildew and anti-wood-decay fungal activities. Research showed that the oil extracted from the leaves was the most effective and that elemol, and alpha-cadinol, were the prominent compounds in producing the relevant activities. This study demonstrates the potential uses of Cedarwood oil in maintaining wood furniture.

Reference:
http://www.ncbi.nlm.nih.gov/pubmed/24273878]

Study 4 – Larvicidal Activity

In this study published in the *Asian Pacific Journal of Tropical Biomedicine*, the larvicidal effects of Cedarwood essential oil were examined, with the following results: "To screen the essential oil of Juniperus procera (J. procera) (Cupressaceae) for larvicidal activity against late third instar larvae of Anopheles arabiensis (An. arabiensis) Patton, the principle malaria vector in Ethiopia...This investigation indicates that J. procera could serve as a potential larvicidal agent against insect vector of diseases, particularly An. arabiensis."

Anopheles arabiensis is a malaria-carrying mosquito. This particular species carries the most lethal form of malaria, with the highest mortality rates and the most complications in treatment. Most of the global malarial infections are in Africa, with over 247 million human infections to date worldwide, 98% of which come out of Africa. 75% of these African malaria cases are the result of the species, P. falciparum, which causes nearly all malaria deaths, with the other strains of malaria being much easier to manage. Malarial symptoms include, nausea and vomiting, fatigue, headache, chills, sweats, and fever.

This study examined the effects of Juniperus procera, or east African cedar, on the An.arabiensis larvae. After 24 hours of observation under World Health Organization standard protocols, the study found that J.procera demonstrated larvicidal activity against the larvae.

Consequently, the study indicates that Cedarwood essential oil can serve as a natural larvicide, combatting the larvae of malaria-carrying mosquitoes.

Reference:

http://www.ncbi.nlm.nih.gov/pubmed/25183156]

http://www.ncbi.nlm.nih.gov/pmc/articles/PMC4025318/pdf/apjtb-04-s1-s099.pdf]

Study 5 – Anti-inflammatory Properties

In this study available on PubMed, the anti-inflammatory effect of several species of Cedarwood essential oil was examined, with the following results: "Ethnobotanical surveys indicated that in the traditional medicines worldwide, several Juniperus species are utilized as anthelmintic, diuretic, stimulant, antiseptic, carminative, stomachic, antirheumatic, antifungal, and for wound healing. In the present study, essential oils obtained from heartwood samples of Juniperus virginiana L., Juniperus occidentalis Hook. and Juniperus ashei J. Buchholz were evaluated for wound healing and anti-inflammatory activities...The essential oil of J. occidentalis showed the highest activity on the in vivo biological activity models. Additionally, the oil of J. virginiana was found highly effective in the anti-inflammatory activity method. The experimental data demonstrated that essential oil of J. occidentalis displayed significant wound-healing and anti-inflammatory activities."

In summary, 3 Cedarwood essential oils – including that of Juniperus virginiana – were tested for their anti-inflammatory and wound healing properties. Juniperus virginiana demonstrated high anti-inflammatory properties, while Juniperus occidentalis, or the Sierra juniper, was found to be effective as both an anti-inflammatory and a wound healer. This indicates the potential for Cedarwood oils in wound recovery and in reducing inflammation.

Reference
http://www.ncbi.nlm.nih.gov/pubmed/23297713]

Study 6 – Antimicrobial Properties

In this study available on PubMed, Cedarwood essential oil's antimicrobial effects were examined, with the following results: "In this study the composition and antimicrobial properties of essential oils obtained from Origanum onites, Mentha piperita, Juniperus exalsa, Chrysanthemum indicum, Lavandula hybrida, Rosa damascena, Echinophora tenuifolia, Foeniculum vulgare were examined...Juniperus exalsa, and Chrysanthemum indicum exhibited antibacterial activities against both Staphylococcus aureus and Escherichia coli. We also examined the in vitro antimicrobial activities of some components of the essential oils and found some components with antimicrobial activity."

The study examined the antibacterial and antimicrobial activities of 8 essential oil extracts – including Juniperus exalsa – against Staphylococcus aureus, Pseudomonas aeruginosa, and Escherichia coli.

Staphylococcus aureus is a Gram-positive bacterium. Although Staphylococcus aureus is part of the normal human skin flora and respiratory tract and is not typically pathogenic, those with compromised immune systems can potentially develop an infection from the bacteria. When it becomes pathogenic, S. aureus produces respiratory issues like sinusitis, skin infections, and even food poisoning.

Pseudomonas aeruginosa is also a common bacteria found in water, soil, skin flora, and in man-made environments. The bacterium thrives on moist surfaces, and can threaten the hospital environment by finding its home on medical equipment, like catheters, resulting in cross-infection. It is, for instance, the bacterium which causes hot-tub rash. This bacterium also attacks immune-compromised patients, infecting the urinary tract, airway, wounds, burns, and resulting in blood infections.

Escherichia coli is a bacterium, as well, though it's Gram negative, rather than Gram positive, like S. aureus. E. coli can often result in serious food poisoning.

The study showed that Cedarwood essential oil was inhibitory against Staphylococcus aureus and Escherichia coli, both gram negative and gram positive bacteria.

Reference:
http://www.ncbi.nlm.nih.gov/pubmed/12510839]

Chapter 4:
The Ins & Outs of Essential Oils

Where do essential oils come from?

Plants and plant species naturally produce essential oils for various reasons, one being to draw pollinator insects to them, another being to repel invading organisms (bacteria, animals). A number of chemical compounds compose each plant's essential oil, and the combination of these compounds are specific to each oil, which then instills in the oil its own unique properties. Essential oils can be harnessed from all sorts of plant components, including flowers, leaves, bark, fruit, roots, and resin. For instance, cinnamon oil is harnessed from bark, lemon oil from the peel, and lavender oil from flowers. Certain plants can produce a few chemical variants of the same essential oil, which are acquired from different parts of the plant. Some of these parts produce a large amount of oil, while others produce just a smidgen. The oil's quality and potency depends upon a number of factors, including the subspecies of the plant, its soil conditions, the time of year and even the time of day you harvest it.

How are essential oils extracted?

Essential oils can be extracted from plants through various methods, including pressing, distillation, solvent and maceration. Let's take a brief look at each:

Pressing Method

Commonly used with citrus fruit, the pressing method extracts the oil through a technique which involves pushing the fruit peels through a press. Oily fruits and plants are best suited for this technique. Orange oil, for example, is extracted from orange skins through the pressing method.

Distillation Method

This technique harkens back to the days of moonshiners, as the same sort of method used to create strong liquor can be used to extract essential oils. Using a still, boiled water and plant materials will create steam which is then cooled by coils and condensed into a combination of water and oil. This combination does not mix, so the oil can then be extracted from it.

Solvent Method

Through a multi-step process, certain plant and flower oils can be extracted using alcohol and other solvents, which extort the essential oil from the plant materials.

Maceration Method

When a "carrier," fixed oil, or lard is mixed with the plant material and set out in the sun, over a period of time, the carrier oil is infused with the plant's essence. Heat sources, other than the sun, are often used to speed the process. Throughout the process, more plant material is added to produce a more potent oil.

How do you use essential oils?

Although some studies about the effectiveness of essential oils are conducted by small companies or even individuals, a number of them are conducted by the food and cosmetic industries. In general, the pharmaceutical industry shows next to no interest in herbal medicine, primarily because there are few options to patent such products. As such, the product's lack of profitability results in a lack of research funding. Regardless, the historical uses of essential oils tell us what we need to know: these oils have been effectively administered for centuries. The therapeutic qualifications of essential oils can be plotted in the survival of the human race across cultures and generations.

Another reason that studies on essential oils have not resulted in much conclusive evidence as to their overall effectiveness is because definitive results are sometimes difficult to prove, as the quality of each batch of oil can vary for a number of reasons. One is that essential oils are impossible to standardize. As mentioned above, even the slightest variance in soil conditions and the time of harvesting – as well as innumerable other factors – will produce a different product quality and potency. In addition, essential oils are often obtained from various species of the same plant; Eucalyptus radiata and Eucalyptus globulus can both be used in the making of therapeutic-grade eucalyptus oil and as a result, they may have slightly different properties and degrees of strength or effectiveness.

Just as there are a number of methods by which to extract essential oils, there are a number of methods to administer them therapeutically. The variety of chemical compounds in each essential oil means that their benefits and applications also vary across the board. Below are a few of these methods.

Topical Administration

Direct application of many essential oils works like a sponge, as skin absorbs chemicals and other things (like sunlight, for instance). Topical application is best when you want to clear up an ailment on the skin's surface, or in the underlying muscle tissue. When applying topically, either massage the oil into the skin, or simply dab on the skin for therapeutic results. Combine the essential oil with a carrier oil for topical use in order to dilute its potency. This is safer, as the oil is very concentrated. Support the body's defenses against rash or muscle pain in this manner, but you should always test a patient for allergies before applying. Adverse effects are produced by natural chemicals as much as synthetic ones; poison ivy, for example.

To test for allergens, place a drop or two on your patient's inner forearm. If a rash develops within 12 to 24 hours, then the patient is allergic. In addition, phototoxicity – sun exposure resulting in an exacerbated burn – may be an issue when citrus oils are applied topically. One must proceed with caution when applying essential oils using this method.

Inhalation Therapy

Commonly known as "aromatherapy," this essential oil application is effective for inner ailments, like sore throat or cold. In a steaming bowl of distilled or sterilized water, add a few drops of essential oil and with a towel over the head, bend over the bowl and inhale. The towel captures the vapors, making the technique even more effective. Essential oils can also be placed in a diffuser, or potpourri, throughout a room to produce somewhat diluted medicinal effects.

Ingestion

When using this method proceed with caution. Direct ingestion of essential oils must be monitored and applied in small doses that are diluted in a tablespoon or more of any carrier oil – olive oil, for example. If unsure of dosage amounts, make a tea with the relevant herb instead. Although the effects of this diluted use may be weaker, this application is a better alternative than an overdose of essential oils.

What are the general benefits of using essential oils?

Replacement for Prescription Drugs

One practical benefit for using essential oils is of course, their substitutive nature; they can replace Rx drugs, which is the ultimate reason to educate yourself on their administration and to begin stockpiling an essential oil supply. One of the potential threats of economic, or social collapse, is the lack of resources, and primarily the inability to procure prescription drugs. As such, finding suitable alternatives should be a priority when prepping for the worst.

Their portability is also a major bonus when it comes to survival prepping. The fact that these ultra-concentrated oils take up little-to-no space makes toting them to a shelter all the simpler should the need arise. Because essential oils are highly concentrated, the application used in most methods of administration requires only a drop or two of oil, which means that a tiny bottle will be long-lasting.

Cheap, but Effective Alternative

Though money may be the last thing on your mind when it comes to prepping for a survival situation (money may even be obsolete in the event of social collapse), it is worth noting that the expense of essential oils pales in comparison to prescription drugs. In fact, whether or not you are forced to survive on essential oils due to a lack of prescription reserves, in some cases, you might consider substituting prescriptions for these inexpensive alternatives regardless. Essential oils are a cost effective, but equally effective alternative to prescription medicine.

No Expiration Date

Another benefit of essential oils is that they do not expire, nor do they have "proper storage" requirements. A number of medicines and medicinal products must be replaced every couple of years; this sets essential oils ahead of the pack when it comes to shelf life.

Versatility

Essential oils also offer great versatility. Apart from providing health benefits, essential oils can be repurposed for household and hygienic applications. For instance, if looking for something that might serve dental hygiene needs in a time of crisis, thieves oil is the go-to essential oil. In order to maintain the skin's health, frankincense and lavender will do the trick; the latter also serves as sunscreen, so it can protect against sun damage as well.

When it comes to the house or shelter, use essential oils to deodorize, which will come in handy in a disaster scenario where things might start to smell bad due to lack of proper utilities and care. For example, after the 2011 tsunami and the subsequent nuclear reactor meltdown in Japan, a nurse named Risa Nakahira used essential oils to deodorize and sanitize putrid public bathrooms in overpopulated evacuation facilities. As relief workers searched for survivors, often wading through debris and decay, Nakahira also deodorized their boots and masks using essential oils. The possibilities of these natural oils are endless.

They are also versatile when it comes to the range of patients they are capable of supporting. The health of everyone from great grandfather to infant baby can be fortified with the aid of essential oils in the appropriate dosage. They even come in handy when supporting the health of livestock or pets. From teething infants to dementia in the elderly, from teenagers with acne to dogs with urinary tract infections, essential oils can serve any patient with nearly any ailment.

Conclusion

Now that you know all about what Cedarwood essential oil can do – where it originates, how it is extracted, its benefits and properties, and the different methods of administration – you can use it confidently to support the body's defenses against health issues, and start to assemble a kit of essential oils for survival. Essential oils can be purchased online, or at your local holistic treatment store.

The various benefits of essential oils and their properties are countless. To build a kit, first focus on acquiring the essential oils which may bear more relevance to specific health issues, or the potential health threats within the surrounding environment. For instance, Cedarwood essential oil will be one of the more crucial oils – along with lemon and cinnamon (eBooks also available for purchase) – when it comes to skin health.

Used as a supplement, or as a go-to for skin conditions, stress disorders, or insect repellant, the application of Cedarwood essential oil in medicine has survived for centuries and will survive centuries more. When it comes down to it, you do not need to rely on pharmaceuticals; essential oils, herbs, and plenty of other natural ingredients can be used to help support the body's natural defenses against any number of health issues, whether ailment or injury.

Essential oils are essential to survival in the case of

viral outbreak, social collapse or natural disaster because, when the SHTF, access to pharmaceuticals will likely either be limited or eliminated altogether. Alternatives to our modern-day standard will equate survival when no other option exists. When it comes to a life-or-death situation, you cannot let your health decline, no matter the state of the world.

DISCLAIMER AND/OR LEGAL NOTICES: Every effort has been made to accurately represent this book and it's potential. Results vary with every individual, and your results may or may not be different from those depicted. No promises, guarantees or warranties, whether stated or implied, have been made that you will produce any specific result from this book. Your efforts are individual and unique, and may vary from those shown. Your success depends on your efforts, background and motivation.

The material in this publication is provided for educational and informational purposes only and is not intended as medical advice. The information contained in this book should not be used to diagnose or treat any illness, metabolic disorder, disease or health problem. Always consult your physician or healthcare provider before beginning any nutrition or exercise program. Use of the programs, advice, and information contained in this book is at the sole choice and risk of the reader.